Legal & Disclaimer

The information contained in this book and its contents is not designed to replace or take the place of any form of medical or professional advice; and is not meant to replace the need for independent medical, financial, legal or other professional advice or services, as may be required. The content and information in this book has been provided for educational and entertainment purposes only.

The content and information contained in this book has been compiled from sources deemed reliable, and it is accurate to the best of the Author's knowledge, information and belief. However, the Author cannot guarantee its accuracy and validity and cannot be held liable for any errors and/or omissions. Further, changes are periodically made to this book as and when needed. Where appropriate and/or necessary, you must consult a professional (including but not limited to your doctor, attorney, financial advisor or such other professional advisor) before using any of the suggested remedies, techniques, or information in this book.

Upon using the contents and information contained in this book, you agree to hold harmless the Author from and against any damages, costs, and expenses, including any legal fees potentially resulting from the application of any of the information provided by this book. This disclaimer applies to any loss, damages or injury caused by the use and application, whether directly or indirectly, of any advice or information presented, whether for breach of contract, tort, negligence, personal injury, criminal intent, or under any other cause of action.

You agree to accept all risks of using the information presented inside this book.

You agree that by continuing to read this book, where appropriate and/or necessary, you shall consult a professional (including but not limited to your doctor, attorney, or financial advisor or such other advisor as needed) before using any of the suggested remedies, techniques, or information in this book.

JASON BENNETT

"I have been a seeker and I still am, but I stopped asking the books and the stars. I started listening to the teaching of my Soul."

-Rumi

YOGA

YOGA FOR BEGINNERS – YOGA BODY POSES TO RELIEVE STRESS, ANXIETY, AND DEPRESSION

JASON BENNETT

Table of Contents

Introduction

Welcome! First and foremost, I want to thank you from the bottom of my heart for downloading my book. My intention in this book is to inform the reader of the history, health benefits, and overall balance yoga can bring to one's life. In this book, you will find a few basic poses to get you started as well as explanations of several different yoga techniques. This book is an excellent starting place for beginners that are new to yoga. However, I recommend you taking a yoga class to become completely immersed in yoga and be guided in a way that can benefit you the most. With that in mind I hope this book provides a lot of value to your life and helps you take your first step towards a better you. With that said and done, let's get started...

Yoga is seen today as a form of exercise meant to strengthen the joints and relax the mind, but this is not the sole intent of the practice. The word yoga is as ancient as they come, beginning in India the word originates from the Sanskrit word "Yuj" which means "Union". (The *Art of Living, Shankar, 2017)* The practice of yoga is meant to be a union between an individual consciousness and the universal consciousness. This ancient form of exercise allows one to experience a happier, healthier, and more peaceful way of living life and therefore may lead to a union with one's self. This book will explore various yoga practices and touch on the surface on the exercises themselves, it is the hope of the author that this will encourage the reader to take a yoga class or two to experience the benefits for themselves.

THE YOGA ORIGINS

The beginning of yoga does not have an exact date or time frame, it does however find its origins in Hinduism; a religion which is widely practiced in India. The earliest record in Hindu scripture to yoga appears in 800- 600 BCE. (Hindu American Foundation, 2016) To understand the importance of yoga in the religious capacity you must understand that in its simplest explanation Hindu belief says that "the Supreme Being or Divine resides within all that exists" and within Hindu texts yoga is said to be "a practice to control the senses and ultimately the mind." (HAF, 2016) In the Hindu texts Yoga practices were determined by four different classifications; *Bhakti* which meant devotion, *Jnana* which meant knowledge, *karma* which meant action, and *Dhyana* which meant devotion. (HAF, 2016) Yoga today is a balancing exercise intended to help cleanse oneself of impurities, to better oneself spiritually and emotionally, and to push yourself physically this was the intent of *Dhyana* in Hindu yoga practice. Unfortunately, the worldwide commercialization of yoga as an exercise has taken away from the importance of the practice as a religious development for further personal growth. While there is no doubt that yoga can help change your body for the better, it should be noted that to truly practice and appreciate yoga the practitioner should also understand and respect the true meaning and intent of the culture that created it.

Chapter 1

HEALTH BENEFITS OF YOGA

Yoga is rapidly becoming one of the most widely used forms of exercise, especially in the Western world. The practice has become popular for those of prominence such as celebrities, athletes, and others in the public eye which has made it increasingly intriguing for the everyday Westerner to use. This has created a spike in the number of yoga classes being offered in schools, gyms, and parks all around the world. There is no doubt that yoga can be an extremely beneficial exercise as it has many benefits.

Improving flexibility

For many who practice yoga their flexibility improves after just a few classes. Many poses are meant to loosen the joints and muscles, allowing for you to get closer and closer to touching your toes after each class. Each pose allows your body to stretch as far as physically possible and allows the joins and muscle a new range of motion that they may not have had before. A body with a greater range of motion is less prone to injury because it can handle some stress being place on it.

Stress Relief

We all suffer from a form of stress in our life, the constant movement and fast pace of modern life has increased people's stress levels immensely. Breathing is an important part of yoga, and when you allow your body even just a few minutes of concentrated breathing with no outside stimulation it will relax and exhale the stresses of your day. As human beings, we spend our days constantly moving and spend very little time trying to quite our minds and bodies, which puts an immeasurable amount of unforeseen stresses on your body. If you do not take the time to release these stresses that have built up from your day to day life you can make your body weaker and more prone to injury. Through the practice of yoga, the mind is quite and with each breath and each pose the stress of your day will melt away.

Improved Immunity

The immune system is our bodies defense from the outside world. Any imbalance in your body can affect the mind, just as any imbalance in the mind can affect the body. Everything is connected; the mind, body and soul. Yoga poses are meant to massage and stretch the internal and external parts of your body which can strengthen your muscles, increase your circulation and detoxify the body. When the mind is cleansed the body is cleansed, and is more able to fight off toxins and outside illness.

Increased energy

The breathing method used in yoga causes the body to slow down and forces it to begin a recharging process that is useful in this hectic world. The breathing method is naturally energizing and can help blood flow, which sends more oxygen to the brain and increasing energy. Getting up for even just a few minutes a day can change your energy level immensely. Yoga will help to elevate your mood and make you feel refreshed and energized.

Weight Loss

Many yoga practitioners are clean eaters and mindful of their overall bodies health. Studies have shown that those who practice yoga have an overall lower body mass index (BMI), many attribute this to the mindfulness. Those who practice yoga are more likely to be mindful of their food intake and what their body needs to thrive. Those who practice yoga tend to be less likely to over eat, and have a more positive relationship with food. With this positive relationship, the practitioner is less likely to be overweight.

Yoga styles

There are many different yoga styles out there today, included are several of these. It should be noted however, that you should try each style and determine what fits your body and needs.

Anusara

Anusara was created in 1997 but John Friend, making it a newer form of yoga than those practiced in India. The practice was created with the basic belief that each human is filled with goodness. This style is used to help the practitioner open their hearts, experience grace, and allow their inner goodness to show. This style of yoga can often be difficult physically at first, after several classes though it becomes easier to adapt to the flow that the teacher creates. (*Gaiam, 2017*)

Ashtanga

Ashtanga yoga is based on the ancient practices of yoga. This style is rigorous and always follows the same movement pattern. This differs from other styles where the teacher can determine which pose will follow another. This style was popularized in the Western world by Pattabhi Jois in the 1970's and has taken off from there. This style can be physically demanding, so it is not recommended as a newcomer's style. (*Gaiam, 2017*)

Bikram

Approximately 30 years ago Bikram Choudhury created a yoga practice that is to be done in heated rooms. Like Ashtanga, this style follows the same movement pattern each time. During this practice, the student will become extremely sweaty and tired, providing a more strenuous workout than some of the other yoga styles. This style has become one of the most popular among westerners, so classes are never hard to find. (*Gaiam, 2017*)

Hatha

Hatha is a term that covers any yoga style that teaches physical postures and movements. Almost every yoga that is taught in the Western world is a Hatha yoga style, making it a generic term. If a class you are taking has "Hatha" in the name, it just means that there will an introduction to the practice of yoga and generally refers to an easier class. Most do not find this style of yoga tiring; however, it is a great start and begins the process of loosen your joints and muscles. *(Gaiam, 2017)*

Iyengar

Iyengar yoga was created by B.K.S Iyengar and is a meticulous style of yoga. Attention is paid to finding the perfect alignment in each pose during the practice. Although this is not the most physically challenging yoga style there is, it can become mentally strenuous. Iyengar classes will usually have yoga props to help the practitioner find their perfect alignment, these could be blocks, blankets, chairs, straps etc. For those with chronic pain or previous injury

Iyengar yoga may be the best practice for you to begin your yoga journey with. (*Gaiam, 2017*)

Jivamukuti

Created by Sharon Gannon in 1984, this practice has integrated some of the ancient yoga teachings with western styles. This style is physically and mentally challenging and integrates the elemental teachings of ancient yoga with a grueling workout. Jivamukuti translates to "liberation while living". Each class also incorporates Sanskrit chatting into the practice. (*Mind Body Green; Ward; 2016*)

Kripalu

Kripalu allows your body to become your teacher. This is a three – part practice that strives to teach you to know, accept, and learn from your body. When you begin a Kripalu class you are first asked to figure out how your body reacts to different poses, it is necessary to listen to your body and not push it beyond its limits in this practice. Poses are held for long periods of time, and a lot of meditation is also incorporated into Kripalu; allowing for your body to focus on its needs. (*Mind Body Green; Ward; 2016*)

Prenatal

Prenatal yoga was created for expectant mothers. However, it can be beneficial during all stages of pregnancy and even after. During pregnancy keeping your muscles strong and fluid is important for the recovery of your body after birth. It is easier to whip your body back in shape after baby if the muscles were worked during pregnancy. (*Mind Body Green; Ward; 2016*)

Restorative

Restorative yoga was created as a style to help the practitioner that experiences nervousness; and creates a relaxing environment that most people in today's hectic world could benefit from. There is little activity in this style, and props are provided so the student does not have to strain themselves to get into a pose. This style is meant to rejuvenate the body and mind, but is not necessarily meant as a form of physical exercise. *(Gaiam, 2017)*

Viniyoga

Viniyoga, or "Vini" means "differentiation", "adaptation", and "application". This is an individualized practice where the practitioner will learn to adapt poses to their own needs and or abilities. This style uses the principles of "proprioceptive neuromuscular facilitation" or PNF. In simple terms PNF means to warm up your muscles before stretching them, which can decrease your chances of an injury during the practice. *(Mind Body Green; Ward; 2016)*

Vinyasa/power

Vinyasa is a Sanskrit word that translates loosely as "to place in a special way", which refers to the sequence of poses being shown in the class. These classes are known for the movement intense practices as well as the fluidity that is needed to do the poses correctly. Teachers usually will play music to keep the class moving and energized and has each class choreographed to allow for smooth transitions. *(Gaiam, 2017)*

Yin

Yin is a quiet, meditative style of yoga. Often called Taoist yoga, these poses are passive and are intended to lengthen your connective tissues in the body. These poses will relax the muscles and allow gravity to do the work. This style will also allow you to practice patience. *(Mind Body Green; Ward; 2016)*

Chapter 2

BASIC YOGA EXERCISES

Downward Facing Dog

Sanskrit name: Adho Mukha Svanasana

1. Begin on all fours, hands and knees should be a shoulders width apart.

2. Move your hands forward and spread your fingers for stability. Press your hips upward to create an inverted "V" with your knees slightly bent.

3. To increase the stretch it is encourage to "walk your dog" by placing your heels to the ground. (*Ortile, 2013*)

Mountain Pose

Sanskrit name: Tadasana

1. Stand with your feet spread hip width apart, and place your arms at your side.

2. Keep your breath slow and deep, at an even pace. Keep your neck aligned with your spin.

3. Take a prayer position, and reach for the sky. (*Ortile, 2013*)

Tree Pose

Sanskrit name: Vriksana

1. Take Mountain Pose

2. Shift your weight to your left leg, and place the sole of your right foot inside the left thigh and find your balance.

3. Place hands in the prayer position once you have found your balance. (*Ortile, 2013*)

Warrior

Sanskrit name: Virabhadrasana

1. Begin with your legs three to four feet apart.

2. Turn your right foot out at a 90-degree angle, and keep your left food in.

3. Keep your shoulders down, and extend your arms to the sides with palms facing down.

4. Lunge into your right knee, keep your knee over your foot and don't let it go over your toes.

5. Switch sides (*Ortile, 2013*)

Bridge Pose

Sanskrit name: Setu Bhanda

1. Lie on the floor, hands at your sides.

2. Knees bent, lift your hips up from the floor by pressing your feet to the ground.

3. Clasp your hands under your back and press up for support. (*Ortile, 2013*)

Child's Pose

Sanskrit name: Balasana

1. Sit upright on your heels.

2. Roll your upper body forward and rest your forehead on the ground in front of you.

3. Extend your arms forward and lower your chest to your knees. (*Ortile, 2013*)

YOGA AND HEALTHY EATING

Many who practice yoga believe that food is the life source for our bodies and brings vitality, energy and overall good health. They strongly believe that everything you eat is food for the soul, therefore the food you put into your body can directly affect the level of conscious development you can achieve. Yoga suggests a "pure vegetarian" diet. Many believe that this facilitates the development of "sattva" which is determined as a quality of awareness, connection, love and peace with all beings. It is the belief for many who practice yoga that the food we eat is the first interaction with the world around us; and if we do not eat with a sense of "sattva" that facets of their lives are bound to suffer. (*The Yogic Diet; Mitchell; 2012*)

Foods to eat:

- Fruits that are naturally sweet
- Vegetables, except for onions and garlic
- Beans and Tofu
- Plant based oils; such as sesame, sunflower and olive oil.
- Whole grains; oats, wheat and rice.
- Herbal teas
- Sweet spices; like cinnamon, mint, basil, fennel etc.
- Nuts and seeds that have not been artificially salted

Foods to Avoid:

- Meat and all fish (including eggs)
- Processed or artificial foods
- Fried foods
- Animal fats

- Alcohol and Tobacco

- Canned foods

- Garlic, onions or spicy foods

- White flour and white sugar

  (*The Yogic Diet; Mitchell; 2012*)

Chapter 3

MEDITATION THROUGH YOGA

Meditation and yoga go hand in hand. To maintain a balanced life, you must be able to quiet your mind and body, meditation is the best way to do this. Most yoga classes will include a meditation to cool the body and mind after your practice has ended.

Steps of meditating using yoga

1. Find a quiet place and seclude yourself for five to ten minutes. Make sure your find a space that you are

comfortable in and that no outside stimulant can interfere with.

2. Sit upright in a chair, not too rigidly though. Remove your shoes and keep your feet slightly apart. If you can comfortably sit on the floor, do so. Keep your palms open on your knees.

3. Close your eyes and be aware of your environment, direct your attention inside to the base of your spine.

4. With your eyes closed, firmly press the palm of your right hand onto your head (think about where the "soft spot" on an infant would be). Raise your right hand about six inches above your head with your palms down. Gently, move your palm and down until you locate energy between your head and hand. You may feel it on your palm whether it's cool or warm.

5. Once you locate the energy, place your hand back on your lap. (you may have to try your left hand, this will depend on which is more sensitive)

6. Sit for five to ten minutes in mental silence. If a thought springs up, just watch it rise and fall.

7. Slowly open your eyes at the end of your meditation and be aware of any changes you may be feeling inside your body or any shift in attention.

It should be noted that this same practice of meditation can be done by laying on the floor and mimicking the same motions. Many find that by laying down the body is more relaxed and the mind is able to flow more openly than when your body is positioned in a seat.

Chapter 4

YOGA AND MODERN MEDICINE

Many in the medical field are beginning to become more accepting of Eastern medical practices and are starting to incorporate them into the Western medicine. Many point out that the ever-growing cost of healthcare and the side effects that many medications cause can be outweighed if more holistic methods are intertwined with scientific practice. Dr. George Hung explains that both Eastern and Western medicine have their benefits and their downfalls, and instead of simply using one or the other that a mixture of the two may be the most beneficial. He points out that not all medications are necessary and a better diet and spiritual lifestyle can overcome some illness, however there are many out there that will require a change in their lifestyle as well as western medication to live a healthy life. It is necessary to keep a balance of both to make sure your body is working the way it needs to, if you take the time to listen to your body it will tell you what it needs. *(The Elephant Journal; Hung; 2015)*

Yoga and Illness

As we have explored throughout this book, yoga is not just a religious practice anymore and its benefits are being seen all over the Western world. Many have taken a page from the book of Eastern medicine to help and dull or even cure their illness. Yoga strengthens the mind, body and soul so its use in helping our body heal itself has little room for doubt. It is important to remember to listen to your body though and if these holistic methods are not working you should see a physician. Several disorders have been improved by yoga and living a yoga lifestyle. The exercises performed in a yoga practice can increase blood flow, reduce stress, and increase your lung capacity.

Some who suffer from Type 2 Diabetes have seen an overall improvement in their health through a yoga practice. By changing their diet to one of "sattva", they can decrease their blood sugars and body weight. This can decrease their need for medications. Those who suffer from high blood pressure can also see amazing changes in their health from yoga. The breathing methods practiced can reduce stress and allow you to maintain a healthy blood pressure level. Those who practice yoga do not just forget the techniques and teachings in the classroom when they leave. The calming methods used in yoga can be used in all settings of your life; like the office, the home, social situations etc. When you slow down and calm your mind through a stressful situation, the body is more likely to get through the situation without causing damage to itself. The breathing exercises used in yoga have helped those who suffer from asthma to get through an attack without causing further stress to the lungs through panicking. (*GreenMedInfo; Ji ; 2012*)

Conclusion

Yoga is intended to help one create balance in their life, and allow the practitioner to recharge from their day to day life. Many forget to take time for themselves and yoga is a way to do this without asking a lot from the person. We should all remember to slow down and reconnect with our bodies and minds, and yoga will undoubtedly allow you to do this. Classes are offered in gyms, classrooms, and households all over the world. Taking a class can be a life changing experience and I encourage you all to give it a try. Yoga is not mastered in one day, but my promised to you is that if you implement yoga into your day to day life you will be amazed at the overwhelming health benefits and peace it provides. Thank you for taking the time to read this book, and I hope I left you a little more enlightened on the practice itself. I wish you much love and I wish you the best on your journey!

-Jason Bennett

If you enjoyed this book then I'd like to ask you for a favor, would you be kind enough to leave a review for this book on Amazon? It'd be greatly appreciated!

Thank you and good luck,

-Jason Bennett

Citation Page

- "The Art of Living" Ravi Shankar, 2017

- Hindu American Foundation, 2016

- Gaiam, 2017

- Mind Body Green; Becky Ward; 2016

- 11 Beginner's Yoga Poses to Help Get You Started; Matt Ortile; 2013

- The Yogic Diet: 10 Foods to Enjoy and Avoid; Lisa Mitchell; 2012

- The Elephant Journal, "Yoga and Modern Medicine"; Dr. George Hung; 2015

- GreenMedInfo; Modern Science Confirms Yoga's Many Health Benefits; Sayer Ji; 2012